THE EVERYTHING SOUTH BEACH DIET 2024

A No-Stress Meal Plan for Weight Loss to Boost Energy and Live Healthy, Including Food Lists for Phases 1, 2, and 3

Marian Elbert, RDN

COPYRIGHT PAGE

TABLE OF CONTENTS

Copyright Page.. 2

Table of Contents 4

PART I: UNDERSTANDING THE SOUTH BEACH DIET
.... 1

What to Look for When Choosing the Right Diet 3

The Rising Popularity of Dieting 4

PART II: THE POWER OF THE SOUTH BEACH DIET 6

Paleo vs. South Beach: A Comparative Overview 6

The Challenge of Dieting Success 8

PART III: SOUTH BEACH DIET CULINARY
CREATIONS AND RECIPES 9

TASTY SOUTH BEACH BREAKFAST RECIPES 10

Homemade Pizza Bagels.. 10

Tuna Salad Sandwich... 11

Egg Salad Sandwich 12

Persimmon Pomegranate Fruit Salad............................ 14

Italian Sub Sandwich 15

Green Goddess Deviled Eggs 17

Blueberry Muffin Tops 18

Avocado Toasts with Olive Relish, Tomatoes, and Balsamic.. 23

Quiche Lorraine 25

Sheet Pan Buttermilk Pancakes 29

TASTY SOUTH BEACH LUNCH RECIPES 32

Three Bean Salad 32

Cucumber Sandwiches.. 34

Lemon Pepper Chicken Breasts 36

Garam Masala Fish Sticks 39

Burger Salad... 41

Buffalo Chicken Tacos 44

Chop Suey.. 46

French Bread Pizza 48

Skillet Cacio e Pepe Tortellini with Wilted Greens....... 51

Paccheri with Quick Sausage Ragu 52

TASTY SOUTH BEACH DINNER RECIPES................ 56

Chicken Skillet Enchiladas 56

Grilled Cheese Sandwich with Mozzarella, Red Peppers, and Arugula.. 58

Shrimp Scampi.. 60

Chicken Enchilada Casserole....................................... 62

Ras el Hanout... 65

Fish Stew with Ginger and Tomatoes........................... 68

Cà Ri Gà (Vietnamese Chicken Curry) 70

Asopao de Camarones y Gandules (Puerto Rican Rice Stew with Shrimp and Pigeon Peas) 73

Summer tabouli.. 76

TASTY SOUTH BEACH SOUP RECIPES.................... 78

Hearty Roasted Vegetable and Chicken Stew 78

One-Pot Chicken and Rice Soup................................... 83

Pasta e Fagioli 85

Farro, Mushroom, and Spinach Soup 89

Chinese Hot and Sour Soup 91

Creamy Tomato and White Bean Soup 94

Parsnip Soup with Leeks.. 97

Cream of Celeriac Soup with Brussels Sprouts Chips.. 99

Lemon Chicken Chickpea Soup.................................. 102

Beef Stew 104

Nilagang Baka (Filipino Beef Stew)......................... 107

Tuscan Bean Soup... 110

TASTY SOUTH BEACH DESSERT RECIPES 113

Moist and Easy Carrot Cake Recipe 113

Molten Chocolate Lava Cake Recipe 114

Butter Tart Recipe.. 116

German Chocolate Cake Recipe 117

Dark Fruit Cake.. 120

Graham Cracker Crust Recipe 123

Apple Pie Recipe.. 124

Soft Chocolate Chip Cookie Recipe with Blueberries 125

Chocolate Coconut Bar Cookie 127

Lemon Tarts 129

PART I: UNDERSTANDING THE SOUTH BEACH DIET

When considering dietary changes, it can be challenging to differentiate between plans that seem similar at first glance. The South Beach diet advocate for lower carbohydrate intake compared to the standard American diet and emphasize increased consumption of fats and proteins rather than merely restricting calories.

The South Beach Diet, created by a physician in 2003, is designed primarily for weight loss. It's a low-carb diet that includes foods like whole grains and legumes and restricts processed or simple carbs high in starches, such as white bread and white potatoes. This diet promotes moderate protein intake and an abundance of healthy fats, specifically monounsaturated fats found in olive oil, nuts, seeds, avocados, and canola oil. It discourages consumption of saturated fats and fatty cuts of meat, favoring leaner proteins instead.

The diet consists of three phases:

Phase One: A strict two-week period that eliminates carbs, alcohol, sugar, and starches.

Phase Two: Reintroduction of whole grains and higher-carb foods until the target weight is achieved.

Phase Three: Maintenance phase allowing any food in moderation. If weight gain occurs, reverting to phase one or two is recommended.

Additionally, the South Beach Diet suggests eating six small meals daily instead of three larger ones. Pre-made meals or snack kits can be purchased from the South Beach Diet website, or followers can use cookbooks with diet-specific recipes.

What to Look for When Choosing the Right Diet

When deciding which diet is best suited for your needs, consider the following:

- Weight Loss and Maintenance: If weight loss is your goal, think about how you'll maintain your weight after achieving it. Strict plans followed by a return to previous eating habits often lead to regaining the lost weight. The Paleo Diet shows promise for long-term consistency and ease of adherence.

- Health and Safety: The South Beach Diet, particularly in its first phase, can have similar risks to the keto diet due to extreme carb limitation and potential ketosis, which might be unsafe for some individuals. The Paleo Diet's focus on nutrient-dense foods is generally easier to integrate into normal life.

- Chronic or Autoimmune Conditions: For managing chronic or autoimmune conditions, consulting with a physician is crucial. However, the Paleo Diet is often seen as a nourishing, therapeutic food plan rich in vitamins and minerals.

There are many low-carb dietary options available, each with its unique benefits and potential drawbacks. When looking for a diet that promotes natural weight loss and maintenance while nourishing the body with nutrient-dense foods, evidence suggests that the South Beach Diet might be the most adaptable and sustainable choice for many individuals. Always consult with a healthcare professional before making significant dietary changes, especially if managing chronic health conditions.

The Rising Popularity of Dieting

With nearly half of Americans dieting at any time, it's no surprise that the South Beach Diet climbed in popularity and remain so today. Of those twenty years old or older, forty-nine percent said they were currently, or had tried to diet within the past calendar year. By comparison, only forty-three percent of Americans reported dieting from 2007 to 2008, and CDC records show that the number attempting or actively dieting has steadily increased over the past decade.

PART II: THE POWER OF THE SOUTH BEACH DIET

The South Beach Diet offers a powerful approach to healthy eating that emphasizes whole foods, balanced nutrition, and sustainable habits. By following the principles of the South Beach Diet, you can create a flexible and nutrient-dense plan that supports weight loss, improves overall health, and fits seamlessly into your lifestyle. Always consult with a healthcare professional before making significant changes to your diet, especially if you have underlying health conditions.

Paleo vs. South Beach: A Comparative Overview

Both the South Beach Diet and the Paleo Diet have unique offerings:

The South Beach Diet:

Created as a weight loss plan by a physician in 2003.

Focuses on whole grains, legumes, and low-glycemic index foods.

Promotes moderate protein and plenty of healthy fats, specifically monounsaturated fats.

Divided into three phases: an initial strict phase, a reintroduction phase, and a maintenance phase.

Suggests eating six small meals a day and offers pre-made meals or cookbooks.

The Paleo Diet:

Emphasizes nutrient density and food quality based on ancestral eating patterns.

Includes lean proteins, fresh fruits and vegetables, nuts, seeds, and healthy fats.

Avoids processed foods, grains, legumes, and dairy.

Allows flexibility with the 85/15 rule, encouraging adherence to guidelines 85% of the time.

The Challenge of Dieting Success

Many diets don't work. While it is difficult to estimate exactly how many diets fail or succeed, in part due to reporting bias, some studies have found that as many as ninety-five percent of dieters either give up or regain weight within the first five years. This means that as little as five percent succeed at long-term weight loss.

The main reason people do not succeed at diets is that they are going on diets that are not practical in the long term, do not fit their lifestyle, and do not teach them healthy habits.

PART III: SOUTH BEACH DIET CULINARY CREATIONS AND RECIPES

TASTY SOUTH BEACH BREAKFAST RECIPES

Homemade Pizza Bagels

Ingredients

4 full-sized plain bagels, halved

1/2 cup store-bought or homemade pizza sauce

8 ounces shredded mozzarella cheese

4 ounces mini pepperoni

Dried basil, for garnish

Method

Preheat the oven to 400°F.

For each half of a bagel, evenly spread 1 tablespoon pizza sauce. Top each with about 1 ounce of cheese and dot with a few mini pepperonis (or just divide the cheese and pepperoni between the bagels). Top all your bagel halves just like this. You should have 8. Lightly sprinkle each pizza bagel with a pinch of dried basil.

Bake them for 8 to 10 minutes, until the cheese is melted and bubbly and the bagels are crispy around the edges.

Tuna Salad Sandwich

Ingredients

1 (5- or 6-ounce) can tuna packed in olive oil, undrained

1/3 cup cottage cheese

2 tablespoons mayonnaise

1/4 cup finely chopped red onion

1 celery stalk, finely chopped

1 tablespoon capers

1 tablespoon lemon juice

A pinch or two fresh dill, chopped

2 tablespoons fresh parsley, minced

1 teaspoon Dijon mustard

2 slices bread, lightly toasted

Lettuce, optional

Sliced tomatoes, optional

Method

In a medium bowl, toss together the canned tuna, cottage cheese, mayonnaise, red onion, celery, capers, lemon juice, dill, parsley and Dijon mustard until combined.

Serve tuna salad on toast, either open faced, or between two slices of bread with lettuce and tomatoes, if you wish. For a low-carb option, serve on sliced lettuce.

Egg Salad Sandwich

Ingredients

1 large egg, hard-boiled, peeled, and chopped (See Recipe Note)

1 to 2 tablespoons mayonnaise, to taste

2 tablespoons chopped celery

1 tablespoon chopped green onion or chives

Pinch curry powder

Kosher salt and freshly ground black pepper to taste

Lettuce

2 slices white, wheat, multigrain, or rye bread, toasted or plain

Method

Mash up the chopped egg a bit with a fork. Mix together the chopped hard-boiled egg, mayonnaise, celery and green onion. Sprinkle with salt and pepper and curry powder to taste. Mix with a spoon.

Toast your bread slices if making the sandwich with toast. Put a layer of lettuce on one slice of bread, spread the egg mixture on top of the lettuce, and put another slice of bread on top.

Persimmon Pomegranate Fruit Salad

Ingredients

3 Fuyu persimmons, peeled, chopped (1/4- to 1/2-inch pieces), seeds (if any) discarded

3/4 cup pomegranate seeds

1 Granny Smith or Fuji apple, peeled, cored, chopped (1/4- to 1/2-inch pieces)

7 to 10 leaves fresh mint, thinly sliced crosswise (stack, then roll them up like a cigar, and take slices from the end)

2 teaspoons lemon juice

1 teaspoon honey

Method

Add all

Keeps for at least a couple of days in the refrigerator, but best eaten same day it is made.

Italian Sub Sandwich

Ingredients

1 large loaf Italian bread

1/3 cup mayonnaise

4 ounces Genoa salami

4 ounces pepperoni

8 ounces roasted turkey breast

6 ounces Provolone cheese

2 cups chopped iceberg lettuce

1/2 cup chopped tomatoes

1/4 cup pickled sliced banana peppers (pepperoncini)

1/4 cup chopped Kalamata olives

3 to 4 tablespoons extra virgin olive oil

2 tablespoons red wine vinegar

2 teaspoons dried Italian seasoning

Method

Cut Italian loaf in half longwise with a serrated knife. Scoop out some of the bread in the top half of the loaf. This will give you more room for toppings and make sure the sandwich doesn't fall apart. Just don't go too deep. You still need it to hold together. (Use the leftover bread to make breadcrumbs!)

Spread mayonnaise on the bottom half of the loaf. Layer the meats and cheese on the bottom portion of the loaf in any order you like. I prefer to the do the cured meats on the bottom, then turkey, and then cheese, but there is no science to it.

Chop the iceberg lettuce, tomatoes, banana peppers, and olives. Add a bed of lettuce to the top half of the loaf (that has been hollowed slightly).

Top with chopped tomatoes, peppers, and olives. Drizzle the vegetables liberally with extra virgin olive oil, red wine vinegar, and Italian seasoning. Bring the two halves of the loaf together and press slightly.

Cut the large sandwich into six evenly sized pieces. Serve immediately or wrap and store for later.

Green Goddess Deviled Eggs

Ingredients

6 large eggs

1/2 medium ripe avocado

3 tablespoons chopped flat leaf parsley leaves, plus extra whole leaves for garnish

2 tablespoons fresh chives, coarsely chopped

1 1/2 tablespoons chopped fresh tarragon leaves

1 tablespoon fresh lemon juice

2 tablespoons mayonnaise

1 tablespoon sour cream

1 teaspoon anchovy paste, or 1 small anchovy, minced finely or mashed with a fork

1/8 teaspoon fresh cracked pepper

Salt and pepper to taste

Method

To hard boil the eggs and ensure you can easily remove the shells, you can either steam them on the stovetop or in a pressure cooker. (You can also cook your eggs using the traditional boiling method, but the results don't always peel easily.)

Peel the eggs and cut them in half lengthwise. Scoop out the egg yolks and place them in the bowl of a food processor along with the remaining ingredients.

Process until smooth. It's ok if there are still some noticeable chunks of green in the filling. Taste and add salt and pepper to your liking.

Scoop the filling into a pastry bag fitted with a large star tip. Pipe the filling into the eggs. Alternatively, you can just scoop the filling with a couple of spoons into the eggs.

Sprinkle the tops of the deviled eggs with extra parsley leaves. Crack some extra fresh pepper on top and serve.

Blueberry Muffin Tops

Ingredients

For the batter

1 1/3 cups (182g) all-purpose flour plus 1 teaspoon for dusting the blueberries

1 1/4 teaspoons baking powder

1/2 teaspoon baking soda

1/2 teaspoon kosher salt

4 tablespoons (56g) unsalted butter, softened

1/2 cup plus 2 tablespoons (135g) granulated sugar

1 1/4 teaspoons vanilla extract

1 large egg, at room temperature

4 teaspoons neutral oil, such as canola or vegetable

1/2 cup low-fat buttermilk, at room temperature

1 1/3 cups (7 1/4 ounces) fresh blueberries, washed and well dried

For the streusel and finishing

2/3 cup (85g) all-purpose flour

1/3 cup (37g) rolled oats

1/3 cup (65g) light brown sugar, tightly packed

1/2 teaspoon kosher salt

4 tablespoons (56g) unsalted butter, melted

1/2 teaspoon vanilla extract

Powdered sugar, as needed for dusting (optional)

Method

In a small bowl, whisk together 1 1/3 cups flour, baking powder, baking soda, and salt to combine and set aside.

Add the butter, sugar, and vanilla extract to the bowl of a stand mixer fitted with the paddle attachment or a large mixing bowl using a hand mixer. Beat together on medium speed until fully combined, smooth, and creamy, about 1 minute. Stop and scrape the bowl with a rubber spatula as needed.

Add the egg and beat together on medium speed until fully incorporated. The mixture may look like it's on the cusp of separating. That's okay.

Add the oil and beat together on medium speed, scraping as needed, until fully incorporated.

Add 1/3 of the flour mixture to the bowl with the butter mixture and beat on low until just combined.

Add 1/2 of the buttermilk and beat on low until just combined. Repeat, alternating the remaining flour mixture and buttermilk, scraping the bowl between each addition. Some dry bits remaining are okay. Do not overmix the batter.

Add the blueberries to the bowl you used for the flour mixture. Sprinkle the remaining 1 teaspoon of flour over the blueberries and gently toss to coat.

Add the coated blueberries to the batter. Gently fold the blueberries into the batter until any remaining dry bits have been incorporated and the blueberries are evenly distributed. Do not overmix.

Cover the bowl with plastic wrap and allow the batter to rest at room temperature for 30 minutes or up to 1 hour. This rest helps keep the muffin tops from spreading too much and creates a better dome on top.

While the batter rests, arrange the racks in the top and bottom thirds of the oven. Preheat the oven to 400°F. Line two large rimmed baking sheets with parchment paper.

To make the streusel, add the flour, rolled oats, brown sugar, and salt to a small bowl and mix. Add the melted butter and vanilla extract. Stir the mixture together until most of the flour mixture is hydrated. There will still be some dry bits.

Using your hands, work the streusel until no dry bits remain. The mixture should be crumbly but able to hold together in a clump when you squeeze it. Squeeze together small amounts of the mixture to form little streusel clumps.

Using a 2-inch scoop, scoop out 6 portions of batter onto each baking sheet. To avoid the muffin tops baking into each other, stagger them on the baking sheet and leave a few inches between each one.

Very gently press (you don't want to flatten them) heaping tablespoons of the streusel on top of each muffin top scoop.

Arrange the muffin tops in the top and bottom thirds of the oven. Bake at 400°F for 7 minutes until the muffin top is puffed and the structure is set. Rotate the pans from front to back and top to bottom. Bake for an additional 4 to 6 minutes until the muffin tops are golden on top, golden brown around the edges, and a toothpick inserted into the center comes out clean (11 to 13 minutes total).

Let the muffin tops cool on the pans for 5 minutes. Transfer to a wire rack to finish cooling. If desired, place a spoonful of powdered sugar in a sifter and lightly dust each muffin top. Serve warm or at room temperature.

Avocado Toasts with Olive Relish, Tomatoes, and Balsamic

Ingredients

1 tablespoon chopped red onion

2 tablespoons lemon juice (from 1 large lemon)

1 tablespoon balsamic vinegar

1 cup cherry tomatoes, halved or quartered

1/4 cup sliced green olives

1 tablespoon drained capers

2 tablespoons chopped fresh parsley

1/4 teaspoon salt

Freshly ground black pepper, to taste

4 slices hearty whole grain, artisan-style bread, or another bread of your choice

2 avocados, halved, pit removed, and sliced

4 lemon wedges

2 tablespoons toasted pine nuts

Method

In a bowl, stir together the red onion, lemon juice and vinegar. Let sit for 5 minutes while you chop the tomatoes. Add the tomatoes, olives, capers and parsley to the bowl. Stir in salt and pepper to taste.

The relish can be made a few hours ahead of serving and kept refrigerated. If making further ahead, wait to add the tomatoes and parsley until ready to serve.

In a toaster, toast the bread until golden brown, or to the desired doneness

Top each piece of toast with slices of avocado (left in slices or mashed with a fork), then sprinkle with salt and pepper.

Squeeze a lemon wedge over each avocado toast. Top with the olive relish and the pine nuts.

Serve the toasts immediately

Quiche Lorraine

Ingredients

1 recipe pie dough or 1 deep-dish prepared frozen pie crust

1/2 pound (225g) bacon (you can use more or less to your taste)

1 cup (235 ml) milk

1/2 cup (118 ml) heavy cream

3 large eggs

1/2 teaspoon kosher salt

1/2 teaspoon freshly ground black pepper, or less to taste

1/8 teaspoon ground nutmeg

1 cup (113 g) grated gruyere or other cheese (cheddar works, too)

1 heaping tablespoon chopped chives

Method

If you are making your own pie crust, roll out the pie dough into a 12-inch round. Place it in a 10-inch wide, 1 1/2-inch high tart pan, pressing the dough into the corners. (If you don't have a tart pan, you can use a similarly sized pie pan.)

Use a rolling pin to roll over the surface of the tart pan to cleanly cut off the excess dough from the edges.

Freeze for at least 30 minutes before blind-baking.

Pre-baking is also called "blind" baking. If you're using a store-bought frozen crust, follow the directions on the package for pre-baking.

If you are pre-baking a homemade crust, preheat oven to 350°F. Line the frozen crust with heavy duty aluminum foil. Allow for a couple inches to extend beyond the sides of the tart or pie pan.

Fill tart pan with pie weights such as dry beans, sugar, or rice.

If you are using a pan with a removable bottom, place the pan on a rimmed baking sheet in the oven to catch any spillage.

Bake for 40 minutes. Then remove from oven, remove the pie weights (the easiest way to do this is to lift up the foil by the edges) and the foil, and set aside.

Set a large frying pan over medium heat. Arrange strips of bacon in a single layer on the bottom of the pan (you may need to work in batches or do two pans at once).

Slowly cook the bacon, turning the strips over occasionally until they are nicely browned and much of the fat has rendered out.

Lay the cooked strips of bacon on a paper towel to absorb the excess fat. Pour fat out of the pan into a jar (not down the drain, unless you want to clog the pipes) for future use, or wait until it solidifies and discard in the trash.

Chop the cooked bacon crosswise into 1/4-inch to 1/2-inch pieces.

After the bacon is cooked preheat the oven to 350°F.

Whisk the eggs in a large bowl. Add the nutmeg, salt, black pepper and chives and whisk a little more. Add the milk and cream and whisk vigorously to incorporate and introduce a little air into the mix – this keeps the texture of the quiche light and fluffy.

Arrange the bacon and cheese in the bottom of the pie crust.

Whisk the egg-milk mixture hard again for a few seconds, then pour it gently into the pie crust.

You want the bacon and cheese to be suspended in the mix, so you might need to gently stir it around just a little. You also want the chives, which will float, to be evenly arranged on top, so move them around with a spoon until you like where they are.

If using pan with removable bottom, place a rimmed baking sheet underneath.

Put the quiche into the preheated oven and bake for 30-40 minutes.

Check for doneness after 30 minutes by gently jiggling the quiche. It should still have just a little wiggle. (It will finish setting while it cools.) Cool on a wire rack.

Eat at room temperature, cold (a quiche will keep for several days in the fridge), or reheated gently in a 200°F oven.

Sheet Pan Buttermilk Pancakes

Ingredients

8 tablespoons (1 stick) unsalted butter, melted and cooled, divided

2 1/2 cup (313g) all-purpose flour

1 tablespoon baking powder

1 teaspoon baking soda

1/2 teaspoon salt

1/2 cup brown sugar

2 cups buttermilk

2 large eggs

1 teaspoon vanilla extract

1 teaspoon finely grated lemon zest

1 cup blueberries, divided

1 cup raspberries, divided

Method

Place a rack in the upper third of the oven. Preheat the oven to 425°F.

Pour 2 tablespoons of the melted butter on a 15x10.5-inch sheet pan. Using a pastry brush, brush the butter on the bottom of the baking sheet and up the sides.

Sift the flour, baking powder, baking soda, and salt into a medium bowl.

In a large bowl, combine the buttermilk, eggs, vanilla, lemon zest, and sugar. Whisk vigorously until combined.

Pour 1/3 of the dry ingredients into the wet ingredients. Fold together using a silicone spatula. Repeat until all the dry ingredients are combined with the wet. Continue to fold until there are no streaks of flour. Mix until there is no dry flour on the bottom of the bowl. Fold in 4 tablespoons of the melted butter. Lumps are fine. Your batter should look like loose ricotta.

Fold in half of the blueberries and raspberries into the pancake batter.

Pour the batter into the buttered pan. Using a silicone spatula, spread the batter around so it covers the bottom of the baking sheet completely and is even on top.

Sprinkle the remaining blueberries and raspberries on top of the batter.

Bake the pancake for 15 minutes. Insert toothpick in the middle of the pancake. If it is free from wet batter, it's done. If not, bake for 5 minutes longer. The top of your pancake should be lightly toasted.

Right after it comes out of the oven, brush the remaining 2 tablespoons of butter on the pancake.

Allow the pancake to cool slightly, approximately 3 minutes.

Cut into squares and serve with warm maple syrup.

TASTY SOUTH BEACH LUNCH RECIPES

Three Bean Salad

Ingredients

1 (15-ounce) can cannellini beans, rinsed and drained

1 (15-ounce) can kidney beans, rinsed and drained

1 (15-ounce) can garbanzo beans, rinsed and drained

1/2 red onion, finely chopped (about 3/4 cup), soaked in water to take the edge off the onion

2 celery stalks, finely chopped (about 1 cup)

1 cup loosely packed, fresh, finely chopped flat-leaf parsley

1 teaspoon fresh finely chopped rosemary

For the dressing:

1/3 cup apple cider vinegar

1/4 cup granulated sugar (more or less to taste)

3 tablespoons extra virgin olive oil

1 1/2 teaspoons salt

1/4 teaspoon black pepper

Method

In a large bowl, mix the 3 different types of beans, the celery, onion (drained of soaking water), parsley, and rosemary.

In a separate small bowl, whisk together the vinegar, sugar, olive oil, salt, and pepper. Add the dressing to the beans. Toss to coat.

Transfer the salad to the refrigerator for several hours, to allow the beans to soak up the flavor of the dressing. Let come to close to room temperature to serve.

Cucumber Sandwiches

Ingredients

1/2 English cucumber, peeled and thinly sliced

1/8 teaspoon salt, plus more as needed

8 slices white bread, such as Pepperidge Farm Very Thin White

4 tablespoons unsalted butter or cream cheese, softened at room temperature

1/8 teaspoon ground white or black pepper

Optional: watercress, mint leaves, lemon zest, dill, chives, or parsley

Method

Line a baking sheet with paper towels and spread the cucumbers on top. Sprinkle lightly with salt and leave for 20 minutes. Pat them dry with more paper towels. Taste the slices, and sprinkle with more salt if they taste bland.

Set bread slices on a cutting board and spread one side of each slice generously with butter or cream cheese. You will need about 1-2 teaspoons per slice depending on the size of your bread slices.

Overlapping them to cover the bread, lay the cucumbers on half of the bread slices. If the cucumbers are very thin, make 2 layers, if thick, make one. The cucumber filling should be about 1/4-inch thick.

Sprinkle the cucumber slices with pepper. If you like, top the cucumbers with one of the optional ingredients. Top with a second slice of bread.

Pressing down firmly, cut the crusts off, and then cut into rectangles, triangles, or quarters. Keep it neat!

Arrange on platters (or a plate) and serve.

Lemon Pepper Chicken Breasts

Ingredients

1 1/2 to 1 3/4 pounds boneless, skinless chicken breasts (about 2 large chicken breasts)

1 1/2 tablespoons lemon pepper seasoning, divided

1/2 teaspoon kosher salt, plus more to taste

3/4 cup all-purpose flour

1 1/2 tablespoons vegetable oil

4 tablespoons unsalted butter, divided

2 cloves garlic, minced or grated

1/2 cup chicken stock

1/3 cup freshly squeezed lemon juice (from 2 lemons)

1/4 cup Italian parsley, chopped

Lemon slices, for garnish (optional)

Method

Place the palm of your hand flat against the top of a whole chicken breast to keep it from sliding around. With the broad side of your knife horizontal to the cutting board, cut through the chicken breast to create 2 thinner halves (cutlets).

In a small bowl, combine 4 teaspoons of the lemon pepper seasoning and the salt. Add the flour to a separate shallow dish.

Season both sides of each of the chicken breasts with the spice mixture. Dredge both sides of the seasoned chicken in the flour, shaking off any excess flour, then lay the dredged chicken on a wire rack or platter while you heat the pan.

In a large skillet, heat the oil and 2 tablespoons of the butter over medium heat. Once the butter is melted, swirl the pan a little to combine the two fats. Once the oil in the skillet begins to shimmer, lay your chicken cutlets in a single layer in the pan. You may need to fry in batches.

Fry the chicken for 3 minutes without moving. Use a pair of tongs to flip the chicken and fry until they're cooked through, an additional 2 1/2 to 3 minutes.

Use your tongs to remove the chicken from the skillet to a platter.

Discard the darkened fat from the skillet. Return the skillet to the stove and add the remaining butter.

Melt the butter in the pan over medium heat. Once the butter has melted, add the garlic. Sauté the garlic in the butter until fragrant, 30 to 45 seconds.

Add the chicken stock and lemon juice and deglaze the pan, scraping up any browned bits from the bottom of the pan. Allow the liquid in the skillet to come to a boil and continue to boil until very slightly thickened, about 1 minute. Season the sauce with the remaining 1/2 teaspoon of lemon pepper seasoning and salt to taste.

Once the sauce has reduced slightly, return the chicken breasts to the pan. Turn them over to coat both sides in the sauce and turn the stove off. Allow the residual heat from the pan to warm the chicken up before sprinkling the chopped parsley over top.

Garnish with lemon slices and serve.

Garam Masala Fish Sticks

Ingredients

Cooking spray

1 pound cod fish fillets

1 teaspoon kosher salt, divided, or to taste

1/4 cup all-purpose flour

1 teaspoon garam masala

1/2 teaspoon cayenne pepper

Freshly ground black pepper, to taste

1 large egg

1/3 cup whole milk

3/4 cup panko breadcrumbs

Method

Preheat the oven to 450°F.

Line a baking sheet with parchment paper or a silicone baking mat and spray with cooking spray and set aside.

Using paper towels, pat the fish dry on both sides.

Cut the fish fillet into 3/4-inch wide, finger-length pieces. Sprinkle the fish sticks with salt.

In a medium bowl, combine the flour, garam masala, and cayenne powder and season with salt and pepper. In another medium bowl, whisk together the egg and milk and season lightly with salt. In a third medium bowl, add the panko and season with salt and pepper.

Working with one fish stick at a time, dip it into the flour mixture, ensuring it is coated evenly. Dip in egg wash next, letting any excess briefly drip off, then coat in the panko. Place on the prepared baking sheet.

Repeat with the remaining fish sticks and make sure all sides of the fish sticks are well coated.

Spread the fish sticks out on the baking sheet in a single layer. Spray the tops with cooking spray.

Bake the fish sticks until they are cooked through and crispy on the outside, 12 to 15 minutes, flipping halfway through baking. They will not be especially brown.

Sprinkle the fish sticks with salt. Serve them warm with a dipping sauce of your choice.

Burger Salad

Ingredients

For the burgers:

1 pound ground beef (90/10 or whatever leanness you prefer)

2 teaspoons burger seasoning or 3/4 teaspoon each kosher salt and ground black pepper, mixed together

Avocado oil cooking spray

For the dressing/sauce (makes 1 cup):

1/2 cup mayonnaise

1/4 cup ketchup

2 tablespoons yellow mustard

2 tablespoons dill pickle relish (or finely chopped dill pickle)

1/4 teaspoon garlic powder

1/4 teaspoon onion powder

1/4 teaspoon ground black pepper

For the salads:

8 cups (about 16 ounces, from one medium head) chopped iceberg lettuce

1/2 medium red or yellow onion, sliced thinly

1 beefsteak or slicing tomato, cut into bite-sized pieces, or 1 cup cherry tomatoes, halved

24 dill pickle chips (or 2 medium-sized dill pickles, thinly sliced)

1 cup shredded cheddar cheese (I like Tillamook Farmstyle Shreds)

Ground black pepper

Method

Divide the ground beef into 4 even portions. Using your hands or a burger mold, shape them into patties about 4 inches in diameter and 1/2" thick. Sprinkle the burger seasoning onto both sides of each patty (1/4 teaspoon per side).

Heat a large, heavy-bottomed skillet over medium-high heat for about 3 minutes. Spray the pan with avocado oil, then add the burger patties. Let them sear for 3 minutes, or until they are well browned and will release easily from the pan.

Use a thin, flexible spatula to flip the burgers. Leave them to cook for 3 minutes more, without moving them around, until they are well seared on both sides and still just a bit pink in the middle (you can cut one open to test, if you like, or use an instant read thermometer and refer to the temperature guide here). Remove the patties to a dish to rest.

In a small mixing bowl, stir together the mayo, ketchup, mustard, relish, garlic powder, onion powder, and pepper until evenly combined.

In four wide, shallow bowls, arrange the lettuce, onion, tomato, pickle chips, and cheddar cheese. (I like to sprinkle each ingredient evenly around the bowl rather than making piles of ingredients, so each bite gets some of everything.) Top each salad with one of the burger patties, then drizzle a few tablespoons of the burger sauce onto each salad, to taste.

Top each salad with a couple grinds of black pepper and serve right away.

Buffalo Chicken Tacos

Ingredients

6 tablespoons (3/4 stick) unsalted butter

1/2 cup hot sauce, such as Franks RedHot or Cholula

1/2 teaspoon garlic powder

1 small or 1/2 large plain rotisserie chicken (about 1 3/4 pounds), shredded (about 4 packed cups)

3 tablespoons whole milk plain Greek yogurt or sour cream

2 tablespoons freshly squeezed lime juice (about 1 medium lime)

1 tablespoon olive oil

1/2 teaspoon kosher salt

1/4 teaspoon freshly ground black pepper

4 packed cups (10 ounces) coleslaw mix

12 (6-inch) flour tortillas

2 green onions, thinly sliced

4 ounces blue cheese, crumbled (about 1 cup)

Method

Microwave the butter in a large microwave-safe bowl in 4 to 6 (10-second) bursts until just melted. Add the hot sauce and garlic powder and whisk until combined. Add the shredded chicken and toss to coat.

Alternatively, melt the butter in a small saucepan over medium-low heat. Turn off the heat and add the hot sauce and garlic powder, then transfer to a large bowl and combine with the chicken.

Place the Greek yogurt or sour cream, lime juice, olive oil, salt, and pepper in a large bowl and whisk to combine. Add the coleslaw mix and toss to coat.

Stack the tortillas on a microwave-safe plate and cover with a damp paper towel. Microwave until warm, 30 to 45 seconds. Wrap the stack in a clean kitchen towel or aluminum foil to keep warm until ready to use.

To assemble the tacos, top the warmed tortillas with coleslaw. Top with the buffalo chicken and garnish with the scallions and blue cheese.

Chop Suey

Ingredients

2 tablespoons vegetable oil

1 pound boneless, skinless chicken thighs, cut into 1 1/2-inch pieces

1/2 medium white onion, chopped

2 medium carrots, cut into 1/4-inch coins

1/3 cup low-sodium chicken broth

2 tablespoons oyster sauce

1 tablespoon soy sauce

2 teaspoons sugar

2 teaspoons sesame oil

8 to 10 shiitake mushrooms, stemmed

1 red bell pepper, cut into 1-inch pieces

2 ribs celery, cut into 1-inch pieces

4 ounces snow peas, trimmed

2 green onions, sliced into 1 1/2-inch pieces

3 ounces mung bean sprouts

1 1/2 teaspoons cornstarch

1 1/2 teaspoons water, to dissolve cornstarch

Salt, to taste

3 cups steamed rice, for serving

Method

Add the oil to a wok or a large, deep non-stick skillet over medium-high heat. Heat the oil just until it starts to smoke, about 1 minute.

Add the chicken thighs. Stir fry until the chicken is no longer pink, about 5 minutes.

Add the onion, carrots, chicken broth, oyster sauce, soy sauce, sugar, and sesame oil. Stir fry over high heat for 5 minutes. The sauce should be bubbling.

Add mushrooms, bell pepper, and celery. Stir fry until the celery has softened to crisp-tender, about 5 minutes.

Add the peas, green onions, and bean sprouts. Stir fry until well-mixed and heated through, about 2 minutes.

Add the cornstarch and water to a small bowl and stir to dissolve. Add the cornstarch slurry to the pan and stir fry until the sauce has thickened to your liking, 1 to 2 minutes. Taste and add salt, if needed. Serve with rice.

French Bread Pizza

Ingredients

1 loaf French bread (about 14 ounces)

4 tablespoons butter, room temperature

3 tablespoons olive oil, plus more for finishing

1 cup canned crushed tomatoes (about 1/2 a 14-ounce can)

2 cloves garlic, 1 finely grated and 1 whole

1 teaspoon dried oregano

1/2 teaspoon chili flakes

Kosher salt, to taste

4 1/2 ounces fresh mozzarella cheese

1 sprig fresh Italian basil

Method

Preheat the broil function on your oven to high and move one rack to the top position, and one rack to the center.

Slice the loaf of bread in half lengthwise, then press each side down with your hands to flatten the surface a bit.

Slice in half crosswise and transfer the 4 pieces to a baking sheet. Spread the exposed bread with butter and drizzle with half the olive oil. Broil the loaf until golden brown, about 3 to 5 minutes depending on your broiler, then remove and set aside.

Turn off the broiler and preheat the oven to 450°F.

Add the crushed tomatoes to a small bowl. Add the grated garlic, oregano, chili flakes, and a pinch of salt and mix to combine. Rip the mozzarella cheese with your hands into large pieces. Rip the basil leaves from the stem and set aside.

Rub the whole garlic clove onto the cut side of each piece of toasted bread. Spread between 2 and 4 tablespoons of tomato sauce onto each piece of toasted bread, depending on your preference for sauciness.

Divide the mozzarella cheese equally over the top of the pizzas and top with a final drizzle of olive oil.

Bake on the center rack at 450°F, until the cheese is melted and slightly browned, 8 to 10 minutes. You can also give them a final blast on the top rack under the broiler, if desired. Just keep a close eye so the bread doesn't burn.

Season with salt (if needed) and let cool for a few minutes before finishing with the basil leaves. Slice into pieces and serve.

If you have any leftovers, wrap them tightly in tin foil and store in the fridge for up to 2 days. Unwrap and reheat in a preheated oven at 400°F until warmed through, about 8 minutes.

Skillet Cacio e Pepe Tortellini with Wilted Greens

Ingredients

5 tablespoons olive oil, divided

2 (8 to 9-ounce) packages fresh cheese tortellini, or 1 (16- to 20-ounce) bag frozen cheese tortellini

1 teaspoon kosher salt

2 teaspoons freshly ground black pepper, plus more for serving

1 1/2 cups water

3 ounces baby kale or spinach (about 3 packed cups)

1 cup finely grated Pecorino Romano cheese, plus more for serving

Method

Heat 3 tablespoons of olive oil in a 12-inch cast iron skillet over medium heat until shimmering. Add the tortellini in an even layer. Cook, tossing occasionally, until nicely browned in spots, 2 to 4 minutes.

Add the water, kosher salt, and black pepper. Stir with a wooden spoon to combine, scraping up browned bits from the bottom of the pan. Cover with a lid or baking sheet and cook, stirring and scraping up any browned bits from the bottom of the pan occasionally, until the pasta is tender and glossy and almost all of the water has evaporated, 3 to 5 minutes.

Remove from the heat and stir in the greens, handfuls at a time, until just wilted, about 2 minutes. Stir in the grated cheese and the remaining 2 tablespoons of olive oil. Serve garnished with additional grated cheese and freshly ground black pepper.

Paccheri with Quick Sausage Ragu

Ingredients

1 pound paccheri pasta

2 tablespoons olive oil

2 tablespoons butter

1 medium red onion, thinly sliced

4 cloves garlic, thinly sliced

1 tablespoon fennel seeds

1 teaspoon chili flakes, optional

10 1/2 ounces spicy Italian sausage, casings removed

1/3 cup tomato paste

1 1/2 tablespoons kosher salt for salting the pasta water, plus more to taste

1 1/4 cup pasta water (you'll reserve it right before draining the pasta)

2/3 cup heavy cream

1/2 teaspoon freshly grated black pepper

Freshly grated Parmesan cheese, for serving

Fresh basil, for serving

Method

Set a large pot of water over medium-high heat. Cover and bring to a boil.

Set a large skillet over medium heat. Add the olive oil and butter. Once melted, add the onion and garlic and sauté until the onion is translucent and slightly softened, about 5 minutes.

Add the fennel seeds and chili flakes (if using) and cook for another minute. Add the sausage, breaking it up in the pan as it cooks. Sauté until the sausage is nearly cooked through, about 5 minutes.

Add the tomato paste and lower the heat to low. Let cook, stirring often, while you start cooking the pasta.

Once the pot of water is boiling, season with salt and add the pasta. Let cook, stirring occasionally, until the pasta is al dente, about 8 minutes. A few minutes before the pasta is done cooking, reserve 1 1/4 cups of pasta water for the ragu.

While the pasta finishes cooking, add the reserved pasta water to the ragu and turn the heat back up to medium. The sauce should be simmering and start to thicken. When the pasta is just about done, add the heavy cream.

Use a slotted spoon to transfer the pasta directly into the pan with the ragu. Gently stir or toss together to coat the pasta in the sauce. Once the pasta is coated and the sauce has thickened up, about 3 minutes, remove from the heat. Taste, adding salt if needed.

Serve immediately topped with black pepper, freshly grated Parmesan cheese, and basil.

TASTY SOUTH BEACH DINNER RECIPES

Chicken Skillet Enchiladas

Ingredients

8 ounces cooked chicken (about 2 cups shredded)

1 teaspoon oil

1/4 yellow onion, minced (about 1/3 cup)

3 cloves garlic

1 (15-ounce) can tomato sauce

1/3 cup water

1 (4-ounce) can mild green diced chilis

2 teaspoons chili powder

1 teaspoon oregano

1/2 teaspoon cumin

8 taco-sized flour tortillas

8 ounces cotija cheese

To serve:

Cilantro

Radishes, thinly sliced

Sour cream

Avocado

Jalapeno

Method

Shred the leftover chicken so it's ready when you need it.
You should have about 2 cups.

In a large, high-sided skillet set over medium heat, add the
oil. Once the oil shimmers, add onion and garlic and cook
for 1 minute, just until softened.

Add tomato sauce, water, diced green chilis, chili powder,
oregano, and cumin. Stir together, then let the sauce simmer
on medium to medium-low while you assemble the
enchiladas.

Put about 2 tablespoons of shredded chicken down the center of each tortilla. (You don't really have to measure the meat. Just divide it evenly among the tortillas!) Sprinkle about 1 tablespoon cotija cheese (just eyeball it) across the chicken, and spoon 1-2 teaspoons sauce over the cheese.

Fold in the sides of the tortilla, roll it up, and put it seam side down in the sauce. Nestle them in the pan. Repeat this until the pan is full. Spoon sauce over the top of the enchiladas.

Sprinkle additional cotija cheese over the top of the enchiladas. Cover with a lid and let them simmer until the cheese is melted and the tortillas look puffy, like they soaked up some sauce. This should take about 5 minutes.

Lift the lid and sprinkle cilantro and thinly sliced radishes over the top. Serve alongside sliced avocado, jalapeño, and sour cream.

Grilled Cheese Sandwich with Mozzarella, Red Peppers, and Arugula

Ingredients

8 slices sourdough bread

Butter, soft and at room temperature

Dijon mustard, to taste

Mayonnaise, to taste

Kosher salt

Freshly ground black pepper

18 ounces jarred roasted peppers (oil- or water-packed), patted dry of excess moisture

12 ounces low-moisture mozzarella, cut into 1/4-inch slices (or shredded, if that's how you roll)

2 cups arugula

Method

Butter one side of each slice of bread. On the unbuttered sides, spread Dijon mustard, mayonnaise, and a sprinkling of salt and pepper. Place two slices of bread (or as many as you can fit), buttered side down, in a skillet over medium-low heat.

Add about 4 ounces of the peppers, 3 ounces of mozzarella, and a good handful of arugula. Press down to keep slightly together, then place slices of bread on top, buttered side out.

Let the sandwiches cook over medium-low heat for about 3 to 4 minutes per side, flipping halfway through, making sure they don't get too browned. After about 6 to 8 minutes total, the cheese in the sandwich should be well melted and the bread toasted. Repeat with remaining sandwiches.

Shrimp Scampi

Ingredients

1 pound (16 to 20 count) large raw shrimp, peeled and de-veined, (if you want, keep the tail on for an attractive presentation)

2 tablespoons extra virgin olive oil

2 to 3 tablespoons butter

Salt

3 to 4 cloves garlic, slivered, or 1 tablespoon minced garlic

1/4 to 1/2 teaspoon red pepper flakes (less or more to taste)

1/2 cup white wine (we recommend a dry white wine, such as a sauvignon blanc)

2 tablespoons finely chopped parsley

Freshly ground black pepper, to taste

1 tablespoon lemon juice

Method

Heat a sauté pan on high heat then reduce to medium high heat. Swirl the butter and olive oil into the pan. After the butter melts it will foam up a bit then subside. If using unsalted butter, sprinkle a little salt in the pan. Stir in the slivered garlic and red pepper flakes.

Sauté the garlic for just a minute, until it begins to brown lightly on the edges, then add the shrimp.

Add the wine and stir to coat the shrimp.

Move the shrimp, so they are in an even layer in the pan. Increase the heat to high and boil the wine for about two minutes.

Stir the shrimp and arrange them so you turn them over to cook on the other side. Continue to cook on high heat for another minute.

Remove the pan from the heat. Sprinkle the shrimp with parsley, lemon juice, and black pepper, and toss to combine.

Serve as is, or with crusty bread, over pasta, or over rice

Chicken Enchilada Casserole

Ingredients

For the enchilada casserole:

4 cups shredded cooked chicken

1/4 cup taco seasoning, homemade or store-bought

1/2 cup chicken stock

1 (15-ounce) can black beans

3 1/2 cups (24 ounces) red enchilada sauce, canned or homemade

24 (6-inch) corn tortillas

16 ounces Monterey Jack cheese, shredded

Optional toppings:

Sour cream

Red onions, sliced

Cilantro, chopped

Pickled or fresh jalapeños

Method

Preheat the oven to 350°F

Lightly grease the bottom and sides of a 9x13-inch baking dish with cooking spray, or use a pastry brush to give the dish a light layer of vegetable oil.

Sprinkle the taco seasoning over the shredded chicken in a medium mixing bowl. Add the chicken stock to the bowl and use a pair of tongs to toss the chicken in the seasonings. The chicken should be evenly moistened and coated with taco seasoning.

Add the drained black beans to the chicken and use the tongs to toss them with the chicken.

Pour 2 1/2 cups of the enchilada sauce into a pie dish or wide, shallow 1 1/2-quart mixing bowl.

Dip 8 corn tortillas into the enchilada sauce in the bowl, one at a time, ensuring each is evenly coated in the sauce. Line the bottom of the prepared baking dish with the dipped tortillas, overlapping them slightly to completely cover the bottom of the baking dish. Sprinkle 3/4 cup of the shredded cheese over this layer of tortillas.

Spoon half of the shredded chicken mixture over the cheese in an even layer. Top the shredded chicken with another 3/4 cup of the shredded cheese.

Repeat the dipping and layering process once more. Top with 8 more sauce-coated tortillas.

Pour the remaining enchilada sauce over the top of the assembled casserole. Sprinkle the last of the cheese over the surface and cover the baking dish with aluminum foil.

Bake the casserole for 25 minutes, covered. After 25 minutes, carefully remove the foil and bake until the cheese is completely melted and starting to brown, another 10 to 12 minutes.

Allow the casserole to cool for 10 to15 minutes. Use a spatula to cut the casserole into 8 squares. Serve the chicken enchilada casserole garnished with sour cream, chopped cilantro, diced red onions, and jalapeño slices.

Ras el Hanout

Ingredients

For the Ras el Hanout spice mix (or substitute a store-bought mix):

1 1/2 tablespoons ground cumin

3/4 tablespoons coriander

3/4 tablespoons ground ginger

2 teaspoons cinnamon

2 teaspoons turmeric

1 teaspoon crushed red chili (for a spicy stew), or 1 teaspoon mild paprika

For the stew:

2 tablespoons olive oil

1 large onion, diced (6 to 8 ounces)

3 tablespoons fresh ginger, grated

2 tablespoons ras el hanout

4 to 5 medium carrots, sliced (about 1 pound)

1 medium parsnip, diced (about 3/4 pound)

2 medium sweet potatoes, peeled and cubed (about 1 pound)

2 roasted red peppers (from a jar or homemade), diced

1 tablespoon lemon zest, grated

1/2 cup dried apricots, roughly chopped

4 cups water or stock

1 (15-ounces) can chickpeas, rinsed and drained

6 to 8 cups baby kale or baby spinach

Lemon wedges, to garnish (optional)

Sliced jalapeno peppers, to garnish (optional)

Chopped cilantro, to garnish (optional)

Vegan or regular yogurt, to serve (optional)

Method

Whisk all the spices together until well-combined. This will make a little more than 1/4 cup of spice mix. Use 2 tablespoons for this recipe, then store the remaining in an air tight container for up to a year.

Sauté the onions in olive oil over medium-low heat for about 5 minutes, until the onions begin to turn translucent. Stir often to avoid browning too much.

Add in the ginger and 2 tablespoons of ras el hanout and sauté for another minute, stirring often.

Add in the carrots, parsnips, sweet potatoes, peppers, lemon zest, apricots, and broth or water, and stir well. Turn heat to medium to medium-high, and cover.

The stew should be bubbling at a low boil during this time. Adjust the heat as needed to maintain a low boil.

Remove lid, add chickpeas, and cook for another 10 to 15 minutes or until parsnips and sweet potatoes are quite soft and just starting to break down. Taste the stew, and add salt, pepper, and more ras el hanout to your taste.

Stir gently until the greens are wilted.

Serve with fresh cilantro, a spoon full of yogurt (either vegan or dairy), sliced chili, and lemon wedges.

Fish Stew with Ginger and Tomatoes

Ingredients

4 small (15 ounces, 443g) red potatoes

2 tablespoons olive oil

3 tablespoons finely grated fresh ginger

1 clove garlic, crushed

1 (14- to 16-ounce, 400- to 453-g) can diced tomatoes

1/2 teaspoon sugar

1/2 teaspoon salt, or more to taste

1/4 teaspoon black pepper, or more to taste

1/4 teaspoon crushed red pepper

3 cups (700ml) chicken stock

2 pounds (0.90kg) boneless firm-fleshed white fish, such as haddock, halibut, hake, flounder, pollock, whiting, or other local fish (it's OK if the skin is still on)

2 tablespoons chopped fresh parsley

Method

Without peeling, slice the potatoes into 1/4-inch rounds. Steam them over boiling water in a vegetable steamer, tightly covered, for 10 minutes, or until tender. Set aside.

Meanwhile, In a Dutch oven or other large pot over medium heat, heat the oil and add the ginger, garlic, tomatoes and their liquid, sugar, salt, black pepper, and red pepper. Cook, stirring, for 3 minutes. Add the stock, bring to a boil, lower the heat, and simmer for 10 minutes, or until the flavors mellow.

Add the potatoes and return the sauce to a boil. Simmer 2 minutes.

Cut the fillets into 3-inch pieces. Add them to the sauce and press them down into the pan to submerge them in the liquid.

Cover the pan and cook for 5 minutes, or until the fish is opaque and flakes easily with the tip of a knife.

Taste for seasoning and add more salt and black pepper, if you like. Sprinkle with parsley before serving.

Cà Ri Gà (Vietnamese Chicken Curry)

Ingredients

1/2 cup coarsely chopped lemongrass, from 2 medium stalks

2 tablespoons coarsely chopped peeled ginger

1 medium yellow onion, coarsely chopped

2 tablespoons Madras-style curry powder, preferably Sun brand

1/2 teaspoon freshly ground black pepper

1/4 teaspoon cayenne pepper, optional

1 (13.5-ounce) can full-fat, unsweetened coconut milk, not shaken

2 tablespoons virgin coconut oil or neutral oil, such as canola

4 large boneless, skinless chicken thighs (about 1 3/4 pounds total), each cut into 3 pieces

1/2 teaspoon fine sea salt

1 1/4 pounds sweet potatoes (white or orange flesh), peeled and cut into 1-inch chunks

3 to 5 fresh cilantro sprigs, coarsely chopped

Method

In a food processor, whirl the lemongrass into a fine texture, about 3 minutes, pausing occasionally to scrape down the bowl. Add the ginger and pulse to finely chop. Add the onion and pulse again to chop.

Add the curry powder, black pepper, and cayenne (if using) and whirl until you have a fragrant yellow paste, about 30 seconds.

Do not shake the can of coconut milk. Open the can and remove 1/3 cup of the thick cream at the top of the coconut milk. Stir the remaining lighter milk, and set both aside.

In a 3- to 4-quart pot over medium-high heat, melt the coconut oil. Add the lemongrass paste and cook for 3 to 5 minutes, stirring frequently, until fragrant and no longer raw and harsh smelling. Lower the heat as needed to avoid scorching.

Add the chicken and 1/2 teaspoon salt, stir to combine, and cook for 1 minute to meld the flavors. Add the coconut milk and a little water to cover the chicken. Bring to a simmer over medium-high heat, cover, and adjust the heat to gently simmer for 15 minutes, stirring occasionally.

Uncover the pot, add the sweet potatoes, and return the curry to a simmer. Continue cooking for 10 to 12 minutes, uncovered and stirring occasionally, until the potatoes are tender.

Turn off the heat, stir the coconut cream into the sauce, and let rest on the burner's receding heat for 10 minutes, uncovered, to blend and mature flavors. Taste and season with salt (unsalted curry powder may require an additional teaspoon), and splash in a bit of water if the flavors are too strong.

Serve immediately, garnished with the cilantro.

Asopao de Camarones y Gandules (Puerto Rican Rice Stew with Shrimp and Pigeon Peas)

Ingredients

1 (15-ounce) can pigeon peas (gandules), drained and liquid reserved

6 1/2 cups water, for soaking the rice

1 1/2 cups rice

1 tablespoon olive oil

4 ounces ham, diced

1 cup medium white onion, diced (about 1 cup)

1/2 large green bell pepper, diced (about 3/4 cup)

1/2 large yellow bell pepper, diced (about 3/4 cup)

1 medium Roma tomato, diced (about 3/4 cup)

3 cloves garlic, minced

2 tablespoons recaito flavor base, store-bought or homemade

1/4 cup tomato sauce

6 stuffed Spanish olives

1/2 teaspoon capers

1 1/2 teaspoons sazon seasoning, store-bought or homemade, optional

1/2 teaspoon oregano

1 tablespoon kosher salt

1/2 teaspoon black pepper

1 pound peeled and deveined shrimp, tails removed

Method

Rinse the rise in a strainer under running water to remove the excess starch from the outside. In a large bowl, mix the reserved liquid from the pigeon peas with the water for soaking. Add the rice to the bowl and soak for 45 minutes.

When the rice has finished soaking, drain the water into a large pot on the stovetop, and turn the heat to medium-low. Keep it at a low simmer; you'll add this liquid to the asopao later.

In a 3-quart Dutch oven or similar large pot, heat the olive oil over medium-high heat. Add the ham and brown it, about 3 minutes.

Reduce the heat to medium. Add the onion, peppers, tomato, garlic, and recaito to the pot and simmer, stirring occasionally, for 6 to 8 minutes; or until the vegetables have softened and begin to form a thick, chunky paste.

Stir the tomato sauce, olives, capers, sazón, oregano, salt, and pepper into the paste, and cook for 2 minutes.

Add the rice into the pot and stir to thoroughly coat the grains in the sauce. Add the pigeon peas and the warmed, reserved soaking water.

Bring the stew to a gentle simmer and continue to cook, uncovered, for 15 minutes.

After 15 minutes, stir the shrimp into the asopao and continue cooking, uncovered, for an additional 5 minutes.

Serve promptly, as the stew will thicken the longer it's left to sit. Thin the stew as needed with hot water or with chicken stock to maintain consistency and flavor, especially when reheating leftovers.

Summer tabouli

Ingredients

135g (¾ cup) burghul

4 roma tomatoes, deseeded, finely chopped

1 large Lebanese cucumber, finely chopped

4 radishes, halved, thinly sliced

1 cup coarsely chopped fresh continental parsley leaves

1 cup coarsely chopped fresh mint leaves

1 lemon, rind finely grated, juiced

1 ½ tbsp. extra virgin olive oil

½ tsp honey

1 tbsp. sunflower seeds, toasted

Method

Place burghul in a heatproof bowl. Cover with boiling water. Set aside for 20 minutes or until softened. Rinse under cold running water. Drain, pressing out excess water with a metal spoon.

Combine burghul, tomato, cucumber, radish, parsley and mint in a large bowl.

Whisk together lemon rind and juice, oil and honey in a small bowl. Drizzle dressing over salad and gently toss until combined. Season. Serve sprinkled with sunflower seeds.

TASTY SOUTH BEACH SOUP RECIPES

Hearty Roasted Vegetable and Chicken Stew

Ingredients

8 ounces baby bella mushrooms, quartered

4 large carrots, peeled and cut into 1/2-inch-thick rounds

1 1/2 pounds Yukon Gold potatoes, cubed (about 5 medium-sized potatoes)

5 tablespoons olive oil, divided

1 1/2 teaspoons kosher salt, divided

1 1/2 teaspoons freshly ground black pepper, divided

1/2 teaspoon harissa powder

4 chicken thighs, skin-on and bone-in (about 1 1/2 pounds)

1/4 cup all-purpose flour

1/2 large yellow onion, chopped

3 large cloves garlic, minced

1/2 teaspoon ground cumin

1 teaspoon ground turmeric

1/3 cup white wine

6 cups (48 ounces) chicken stock

2 bay leaves

3 large kale leaves (any variety), stripped from the stem and torn

Method

Preheat the oven to 425°F

Spread chopped mushrooms, carrots, and potatoes on a baking sheet in three separate rows, keeping each vegetable separate from the others—this will come in handy later when you have to add them to the soup in separate steps.

Drizzle 3 tablespoons of olive oil over the vegetables, then sprinkle with 3/4 teaspoon of salt, 3/4 teaspoon freshly ground pepper, and 1/2 teaspoon harissa. Toss each individual row to coat.

Roast veggies in oven for 20 to 25 minutes. When they are fork tender, set them aside while you finish the soup base. (Note: You don't actually want the veggies to brown too much for this recipe; you want the colors to stay vibrant.)

While the vegetables roast, cook the chicken and begin assembling the stew.

Heat 2 tablespoons oil in Dutch oven or large heavy-bottomed soup pot set over medium heat. Trim the chicken of excess fat and skin. Sprinkle the four chicken thighs with 3/4 teaspoon salt and 3/4 teaspoon freshly ground pepper.

Once the oil begins to shimmer, add the thighs skin side down. Cook the thighs for 7 minutes, until the skin has a nice golden brown color.

Flip the chicken and cook for another 5 minutes. A few bits of skin may stick to the pan when you flip. That's ok.

After cooking, the skin should be crisp and golden, and you should have about a 1/4 cup of fat in the pan. (Just eyeball it; you'll be fine!) The chicken will not be completely cooked, which is ok; transfer it to a plate.

Sprinkle 1/4 cup all-purpose flour over the chicken fat. Use a sturdy wooden spoon to stir continuously and scrape the brown bits (the fond) off the bottom of the pan.

Continue cooking until the color deepens and it looks like golden paste, about 6 minutes. This is the roux that will thicken your soup.

Add the chopped onion, minced garlic, turmeric, and cumin to the pan with the roux. Continue to stir and scrape the bottom of the pan. The roux will get crumbly, and the color will continue to deepen. That's ok.

Keep stirring and scraping the bottom of the pan for about 5 minutes until the onions are cooked through.

Slowly add 1/3 cup of white wine, scraping the bottom of the pan to release any brown bits, and stir for another minute.

Slowly pour in the stock, you guessed it, while stirring! Add the bay leaves and bring it to a gentle simmer.

Remove the skin from the chicken thighs and discard. Add the thighs to the pot of simmering stock.

Cover with a lid, but leave it slightly ajar. Continue to simmer over medium low heat for 25 minutes, stirring occasionally. Don't let it boil.

Use tongs to remove bay leaves and chicken from the pot and transfer to a plate.

Add half of the roasted potatoes and half of the carrots to the pot (reserve the mushrooms). Use an immersion blender to puree the vegetables into the soup.

After pureeing, add the remaining vegetables, including all of the mushrooms, and let them warm through.

When the chicken has cooled enough to handle, use two forks to shred it into bite-sized pieces. Discard the bones. Add the chicken back to the pot.

Stir in the kale. Let everything warm through over low heat for a couple of minutes and make sure the kale is wilted.

Ladle into bowls and serve with fresh crusty bread.

One-Pot Chicken and Rice Soup

Ingredients

2 bone-in chicken breasts, skin removed (1 to 1 1/2 pounds)

1 cup long-grain white rice, like basmati

2 ribs celery, diced small

2 medium carrots, peeled and diced small

1 onion, diced small

2 cloves garlic, peeled but left whole

1 teaspoon salt, plus more to taste (see Recipe Note)

1/2 teaspoon ground black pepper

2 quarts unsalted or low-sodium chicken stock

Juice of 1/2 lemon (about 3 tablespoons)

Chopped fresh parsley, for serving

Method

Combine the chicken, white rice, celery, carrots, onions, garlic, salt, and pepper in a large pot. Add the chicken stock and bring to a boil over high heat.

Once the soup is boiling, reduce the heat to keep the soup at a gentle simmer.

As the soup simmers, skim off any foam that collects on the surface with a spoon. Continue to simmer until the rice and vegetables are tender, about 25 minutes. Remove the soup from heat.

Remove the chicken and garlic cloves using a slotted spoon or tongs. Transfer the chicken breasts to a bowl and shred with two forks. Discard the bones. Return the shredded chicken to the pot.

Smash the garlic cloves into a paste against a cutting board using a fork or the flat of your knife. Stir the paste back into the soup.

Stir the lemon juice into to the soup, and taste. The soup should taste rich, barely salty, and with just a hint of lemon. Add more salt or lemon juice as needed until it tastes good to you.

Divide among bowls and sprinkle with some parsley for serving.

Pasta e Fagioli

Ingredients

3 tablespoons extra virgin olive oil

1 cup chopped onion

1 large carrot, peeled and chopped

1 large celery rib, chopped

2 large cloves garlic, minced

1/4 teaspoon chili flakes

1 teaspoon Italian seasoning

6 cups chicken stock (or vegetable stock for a vegetarian option)

1 cup peeled tomatoes, fresh or canned

1/2 pound ditalini pasta

2 (15-ounce) cans cannellini or borlotti beans, drained and rinsed (or 3 1/2 cups freshly cooked beans)

1/4 cup chopped parsley

Kosher salt and freshly ground black pepper, to taste

Method

Heat the olive oil in a large pot over medium-high heat. Sauté the onion, carrot and celery for 2 to 3 minutes, until it's soft and translucent. Add the garlic, chili flakes and Italian seasoning and sauté another minute.

Add the chicken stock and tomatoes and bring to a boil. Add the pasta and keep the soup at a strong simmer.

When the pasta is al dente, add the beans and cook another 2 to 3 minutes. Turn off the heat and stir in the parsley. Add salt and black pepper to taste.

Lemon Chicken Soup (Avgolemono)

Ingredients

1 pound 2 ounces (500g) skinless chicken thighs on the bone

1/2 small white onion, finely chopped

2 fat cloves garlic, minced

1 small celery stalk, finely chopped

1 medium carrot, finely chopped

3/4 teaspoon ground cinnamon

1/4 teaspoon ground turmeric

2 bay leaves

3 1/4 cup (750ml) chicken stock

4 cups (960ml) just-boiled water, divided

Scant 1/2 cup (90g) short or medium-grain white rice, rinsed

3 1/2 ounces (100g) kale, stalks removed, leaves shredded

3 extra large eggs

1 teaspoon finely grated un-waxed lemon zest

6 tablespoons lemon juice, or to taste

1 to 2 tablespoons chopped dill, or to taste

Extra virgin olive oil

Salt and black pepper

Method

Place the chicken, onion, garlic, celery, carrot, cinnamon, turmeric, bay leaves, stock, and 2 cups (480 ml) hot water in a large saucepan. Season with 1 teaspoon salt and 1/2 teaspoon black pepper. Bring to a boil, then lower the heat, cover, and simmer for 40 minutes, until the chicken is cooked.

Spoon out the bay leaves and chicken and set aside on a plate to cool. Add the rice to the soup with remaining 2 cups (480ml) hot water. Cover and cook for 10 minutes. Meanwhile, use your hands to shred the chicken meat from the bones into very small pieces.

After the rice has cooked, add the kale and return the chicken to the pot. Simmer for 5 minutes, then take off the heat.

In a separate medium sized bowl, whisk together the eggs, lemon zest, and lemon juice until the mixture is foamy with no streaks remaining.

Pour 2 ladles of broth from the saucepan into a cup. Then grab a whisk and slowly add this broth to the bowl of lemony eggs, a couple of tablespoons at a time, whisking constantly.

Don't pour in too much hot broth too quickly, or you'll end up with scrambled eggs. Increase to a steady stream once you are halfway through, still whisking, until you've incorporated all of it. Slowly drizzle the mixture back into the saucepan, whisking the soup constantly as you do so and incorporating it slowly.

Return the pot to low heat, add the dill, and cook for 5 minutes to allow the soup to thicken. Don't let it come up to more than a gentle simmer and, if it starts to look a bit too thick, simply loosen it with a bit of hot water.

Finally, taste and adjust the seasoning, adding a bit more lemon juice, herbs, salt, or black pepper to taste. Serve in warmed bowls with a drizzle of extra-virgin olive oil.

Farro, Mushroom, and Spinach Soup

Ingredients

3 tablespoons olive oil

2 pounds mixed mushrooms, sliced (such as white mushrooms, crimini, Portobello or shiitake)

1 teaspoon dried thyme

2 tablespoons low-sodium soy sauce

2 bunches scallions, thinly sliced

1 1/4 cups pearled (quick-cooking) farro 6 ounces)

1/2 cup white wine

Salt and pepper, to taste

3 cups chicken stock or vegetable stock

4 large handfuls baby spinach leaves

1/2 cup Parmesan, freshly grated

1/2 cup fresh parsley, chopped

Extra Parmesan (for garnish)

Method

In a stockpot or large saucepot over medium-high heat, heat the oil. Add the mushrooms and cook, stirring often, for 10 minutes, or until the mushrooms release their juices and turn golden brown.

Stir in the thyme, soy sauce, and scallions, and cook for 2 minutes longer.

Reduce the heat to low, cover the pot and cook for 10 minutes, or until the farro is tender (taste one of the grains to check). Uncover, turn the heat up to high, and cook for 2 to 3 minutes to reduce the liquid to the consistency of a thick stew. (If the farro looks dry, add a little more stock at this point.)

Cook for 30 seconds, or until the spinach wilts. Stir in the 1/2 cup Parmesan.

Taste, and season with more salt and pepper, if you like. Ladle into bowls and sprinkle a little Parmesan on top.

Chinese Hot and Sour Soup

Ingredients

6 dried Chinese black fungus

6 dried wood ear, black, cloud, straw, or shiitake mushrooms, or one bunch of fresh enoki mushrooms

5 dried lily buds

1 (8 ounce) can bamboo shoots

2 tablespoons red wine vinegar

1 tablespoon white vinegar or rice vinegar

1 1/2 tablespoons soy sauce

1 tablespoon cornstarch

4 cups chicken broth

1/2 block firm tofu, diced into small cubes

1 large egg, beaten

1 teaspoon sesame oil

3 scallions, diced

1/4 teaspoon kosher salt

1 1/2 teaspoons freshly ground white pepper

1/4 teaspoon chili oil (optional)

Cilantro (optional)

Method

Pour boiling water over the mushrooms to cover and allow them to soak for 20 minutes, turning the mushrooms over occasionally. It may not seem like a lot but they will grow quite a bit.

After soaking remove any woody ends with a knife. Cut mushrooms into strips. Reserve 1/4 cup of the liquid and mix with the cornstarch. (If using fresh enoki mushrooms set aside as they do not need to soak.)

Pour boiling water over the lily buds to cover and allow to sit for 15 minutes. Cut the buds crosswise, then tear them up into a few bunches.

Mix the vinegars and soy sauce together and set aside. Open the can of bamboo shoots, drain well, and cut the shoots lengthwise into strips.

Place the chicken broth into a pot and bring to a boil over high heat. Add the tofu, mushrooms, lily buds, bamboo shoots, vinegar mixture, and cornstarch mixture. Mix and bring back to a boil. Once it comes to a boil remove from heat.

Pour the egg in a slow steam while stirring the soup allowing it to instantly cook and feather into the soup.

Add the scallions, white pepper, sesame oil, and chili oil (if using)

Taste and adjust white pepper, vinegar, and salt to taste. Add cilantro (if using) to garnish and for added flavor. Serve immediately.

Creamy Tomato and White Bean Soup

Ingredients

For the soup:

2 tablespoons olive oil

1 large onion, chopped

2 medium cloves garlic, thinly sliced

3 pounds ripe plum (Roma) tomatoes, cut into 1-inch pieces (or two 28-ounce cans whole tomatoes and their juices, crushed in a bowl)

1 (15-ounce) can cannellini beans, drained and rinsed, or homemade

1 sprig fresh rosemary

1 1/2 cups water, plus more as needed

1/2 cup freshly grated Parmesan

1 teaspoon kosher salt, plus more to taste

1/8 teaspoon freshly ground black pepper, plus more to taste

For the garnish:

12 cherry tomatoes, sliced or quartered

1 tablespoon olive oil

1 teaspoon red wine vinegar

Kosher salt and freshly ground black pepper, to taste

12 basil leaves, thinly sliced

Method

Heat the oil in a soup pot over medium heat. Add the onion and garlic. Cook, stirring occasionally, for 6 to 8 minutes, or until softened.

Add the fresh or canned tomatoes, rosemary, beans, 1 1/2 cups of water, salt, and pepper to the pot. Bring to a simmer and cook, uncovered, for 20 minutes, or until the tomatoes are very soft. Remove the rosemary sprig. Stir in the Parmesan.

In 2- to 3-cup batches, puree the soup in a blender until smooth, or use an immersion blender. (Warning! The soup is hot! To puree hot liquid in a blender, only fill it 1/3 full. Cover the lid with a folded dishtowel and hold it down with your hand. Start on low speed, and increase the speed gradually.)

Transfer the soup to a pot and stir in enough additional water to bring the soup to your desired consistency (up to 2 1/2 cups of water). Taste and add salt and pepper, if you like. Reheat over low heat until hot.

In a bowl, stir together the tomatoes, oil, vinegar, salt, and pepper. Just before serving, stir in the basil.

Ladle the soup into bowls, and top each bowl with the fresh tomato garnish.

Parsnip Soup with Leeks

Ingredients

2 tablespoons butter

3 leeks, white and pale green parts only, sliced lengthwise, cleaned, sliced crosswise into 1/4-inch slices (about 3 cups of sliced leeks)

1 1/2 to 2 pounds parsnips, peeled and chopped

2 tablespoons extra virgin olive oil, plus more for garnish

1 to 2 teaspoons kosher salt

4 cups chicken stock (use vegetable stock for vegetarian option)

2 cups water

2 strips lemon zest, 1 x 2 inches each

2 cups finely chopped fresh parsley (reserve a little for garnish)

1 tablespoon lemon juice

Freshly ground black pepper, to taste

Method

Heat butter in a 4- to 6-quart pot on medium heat. Add the chopped leeks, toss to coat with the butter. When the leeks are heated enough that they begin to sizzle in the pan, lower the heat to low and cover the pan. Cook until soft, but don't let the leeks brown.

Add the parsnips and olive oil, and toss to coat. Sprinkle on the salt. Add the stock and water. Add the strips of lemon zest.

Bring to a boil and reduce to a low simmer. Cover and cook until the parsnips are completely tender, at least 30 minutes.

After removing the zest and adding the parsley, puree by using an immersion blender or by working in batches with a stand-up blender. If using a standing blender, fill the bowl no more than halfway, hold the cover on the blender bowl, and start blending at the lowest speed. Return the pureed soup to the pot.

Stir in lemon juice and season with salt, if needed.

Garnish with freshly ground black pepper, a little olive oil, and chopped parsley or chives.

Cream of Celeriac Soup with Brussels Sprouts Chips

Ingredients

For the Brussels sprouts chips:

10 brussels sprouts

1 tablespoon extra-virgin olive oil

1/8 teaspoon sea salt, plus more to taste

For the soup:

2 tablespoons grapeseed or extra virgin olive oil

2 cups diced yellow onion

2 teaspoons minced garlic (from 2 cloves)

1 teaspoon sea salt, plus more to taste

1 medium head cauliflower, cut into florets (See How to Cut and Core Cauliflower)

3 cups peeled and diced celeriac (from 1 large root)

8 cups vegetable broth, plus more as needed

1/4 cup blanched slivered almonds

1/8 teaspoon freshly ground black pepper, plus more to taste

Method

Preheat the oven to 350F. Line a baking sheet with parchment paper or a silicone liner.

Slice the bottom tip of each sprout, and peel off the outer leaves. Trim off a bit more of the bottom, and peel off the next layer of leaves. Continue this process until you've removed all of the leaves.

Toss the leaves with the olive oil and salt, and spread them out in a single layer on the baking sheet. Roast for about 10 minutes, until the leaves are browned and crisp.

Set aside until needed.

While the Brussel sprouts chips are roasting, start the soup. In a large saucepan, warm the oil over medium heat and sauté the onion, garlic, and 1/4 teaspoon of salt for about 5 minutes, until the onions are soft and translucent. Add the cauliflower and celeriac, and sauté for another minute.

Add the vegetable broth and 1/2 teaspoon of the salt, increase the heat to high, and bring just to a boil. Reduce the heat to medium-high and simmer for 20 to 30 minutes, until the cauliflower and celeriac are just tender.

Remove the pan from the heat and stir in the almonds. Allow the soup to cool slightly for 10 minutes. (This gives the nuts time to soften.)

Pour the soup into your blender in batches and puree on high for 30 to 60 seconds, until smooth and creamy. Return the soup to the saucepan and warm it over low heat. Stir in the remaining 1/4 teaspoon the salt, and add the pepper. Season with additional salt and pepper, to taste.

Ladle portions of the soup into bowls, and top with the Brussels sprouts chips.

Lemon Chicken Chickpea Soup

Ingredients

1 1/4 pounds boneless skinless chicken thighs, cut into 1-inch pieces

1 teaspoon salt

1 teaspoon ground turmeric

1 teaspoon ground cumin

1/2 teaspoon ground black pepper

2 tablespoons extra virgin olive oil

1 onion, chopped (about 1 1/2 cups)

1 celery rib, chopped (about 1/3 cup)

4 cloves garlic, minced (about 1 1/2 tablespoons)

1 teaspoon fresh ginger, grated (or powdered ginger)

2 bay leaves

6 cups chicken stock

2-3 strips lemon zest from one lemon

2 tablespoons lemon juice

1/3 cup basmati rice

1 15-ounce can chickpeas, drained, or 1 1/2 cups cooked chickpeas

Cilantro or parsley for garnish

Method

Whisk the salt, turmeric, cumin, and black pepper together in a medium bowl. Add the chicken pieces and toss with the spices to coat.

Heat olive oil in a large, thick-bottomed soup pot on medium high. Add the chicken pieces and brown lightly on all sides, 5-7 minutes total. Remove chicken to a bowl and set aside.

Add the chopped onion and celery to the pot. Sauté until lightly browned, about 5 to 6 minutes. Add the garlic and ginger and cook a minute more.

Add chicken stock, bay leaves, lemon zest strips, then simmer

Add the chicken pieces back to the pot. Add the stock, bay leaves, lemon zest strips. Bring to a simmer and simmer for 15 minutes.

Add the rice, chickpeas, and lemon juice. Bring to a simmer and cook for 20 minutes, until the rice is cooked through.

Remove bay leaves and lemon peel strips. Add salt and pepper to taste. Garnish with cilantro or parsley to serve.

Beef Stew

Ingredients

3 pounds well-marbled beef chuck stew meat, cut into 1-inch pieces

1 tablespoon plus 1 teaspoon kosher salt, divided, plus more to taste

3 tablespoons olive oil

5 ribs celery, cut into 1-inch pieces (about 2 cups)

1 medium onion, chopped (about 1 cup)

4 medium carrots, peeled and cut into 1-inch pieces (about 2 cups)

2 medium parsnips, peeled and cut into 1-inch pieces (about 1 cup)

1/2 teaspoon freshly ground black pepper

1 tablespoon finely chopped fresh thyme leaves

1 tablespoon all-purpose flour

4 cups beef broth

2 cups water

1 tablespoon balsamic vinegar

1 tablespoon Worcestershire sauce

1 1/2 pounds russet potatoes, peeled, cut into 1-inch pieces (about 3 cups)

1/4 cup chopped fresh parsley leaves

Method

In a large bowl, season the beef pieces with 1 tablespoon of the salt. Heat the olive oil in a large (6 to 8 quart), thick-bottomed pot over high heat.

Add the beef all at once and cook, stirring occasionally, until the meat is no longer pink and some liquid has accumulated at the bottom of the pot, about 10 minutes.

Add the celery, onion, carrots, and parsnips. Reduce heat to medium-high. Season with remaining teaspoon of salt and 1/2 teaspoon pepper. Cook, stirring occasionally, until most of the liquid has evaporated and vegetables are slightly softened, about 10 minutes more.

Add the thyme and flour, stir, and cook until raw flour is no longer visible, about 30 seconds.

Add the beef broth, water, balsamic vinegar, and Worcestershire sauce. Bring mixture to a boil, then reduce heat to medium-low and cook, partially covered and stirring every 20 minutes or so, until stew has darkened and thickened slightly, about 1 hour.

Add potatoes to the stew, stir well, and continue to simmer until the potatoes and beef are tender, about 30 minutes.

Season to taste, transfer to serving bowls, sprinkle with parsley, and serve.

Nilagang Baka (Filipino Beef Stew)

Ingredients

2 pounds beef chuck stew meat (cubed), or beef sirloin, cubed

2 pounds beef short ribs

1 teaspoon baking soda

2 tablespoons vegetable oil

1 large white or yellow onion, chopped

2 cloves garlic, minced

2 green onions, chopped, white and green parts separated

10 cups water, or enough to fully cover the meats and vegetables

1 tablespoon fish sauce, like Red Boat

2 medium yellow or white potatoes, (5 to 10 ounces each), peeled and quartered

1 medium carrot (about 3 ounces), peeled and sliced

8 ounces green beans, trimmed and cut into 2-inch pieces (about 2 cups)

1/4 pound green cabbage, cut into 8 wedges

1/2 teaspoon kosher salt

1/4 teaspoon ground black pepper

For serving

4 cups steamed rice, optional

1/4 cup fish sauce

Method

Wash the beef in cold water. Pat dry with paper towels.

Add the beef stew cubes and the beef short ribs to a large mixing bowl. Sprinkle the baking soda all over the meat, making sure to spread all around evenly. Let the baking soda marinate for 30 minutes. This will help tenderize the meat.

After exactly 30 minutes, wash off the baking soda from the beef cubes and pat dry with paper towels. Set aside.

Add the oil to a large stockpot over medium heat. When the oil is hot, add the onion, garlic, and white scallions and sauté until fragrant, about 2 minutes.

Add the beef followed by the water. Add the fish sauce and stir to combine. Cover and cook over medium heat, simmering the beef until soft and tender, about 2 hours. Pierce the beef with a fork—it should be fall off the bone tender.

Add the potatoes and carrots and stir. Continue cooking until the vegetables are tender, about 15 to 20 minutes. Add the green beans and cabbage and mix well.

Cover the pot and continue cooking until the greens are tender, about 10 minutes.

Season with salt and pepper.

Ladle the meat, vegetables, and broth into a large tureen or soup bowl. Sprinkle the scallion greens on top for garnish. Serve piping hot with steamed rice and a side of fish sauce.

Tuscan Bean Soup

Ingredients

For the soup:

3 tablespoons olive oil

2 medium carrots, thickly sliced

1 large onion, coarsely chopped

1 rib celery, coarsely chopped

1 clove garlic, finely chopped

3 sprigs fresh oregano

1/4 teaspoon salt

Black pepper, to taste

2 (15-ounce) cans cannellini beans, or other small white beans, drained and rinsed

5 cups chicken stock or vegetable stock

4 cups baby kale or baby spinach, stems removed if tough

1 tablespoon chopped fresh oregano, for garnish

Olive oil, to serve

Extra grated Parmesan, to serve

For the parmesan toasts:

1/2 baguette, thinly sliced

Olive oil

1/2 cup grated Parmesan

Method

In a soup pot, heat the olive oil. When it is hot, add the carrots, onion, celery, garlic, fresh oregano sprigs, salt, and pepper. Cook, stirring often, for 10 minutes until the vegetables look softened and the onions turn translucent.

On a plate, mash 1/2 cup of the beans with a fork or potato masher. Add them to the vegetables in the pot. Cook, stirring, for 2 minutes.

Add the remaining beans to the pot and stir well. Stir in the chicken stock and bring to a boil. Lower the heat, partially cover with the lid placed askew, and simmer for 20 minutes, or until the carrots are tender and the liquid is flavorful.

Discard the oregano sprigs; the leaves will have fallen into the soup. Add additional salt and pepper to taste.

Toast the bread until lightly golden on both sides. While the toast is still hot from the toaster, sprinkle with olive oil and cheese. If you have a toaster oven, return them to the toaster for 1 minute to melt the cheese; otherwise, arrange the toasts in a skillet over medium heat, cover, and warm for about 1 minute or until the cheese has melted.

Add the kale or spinach to the pot and simmering for another 2 minutes, or just until the greens wilt.

Ladle the soup into bowls, sprinkle with oregano and more olive oil, if you like. Serve with Parmesan toasts and extra Parmesan for sprinkling.

TASTY SOUTH BEACH DESSERT RECIPES

Moist and Easy Carrot Cake Recipe

Ingredients

1 1/2 cups oil

2 cups sugar

4 eggs

2 cups all-purpose flour

2 teaspoons baking powder

2 teaspoons allspice, or cinnamon

1 pinch salt

1 larger can crushed pineapple

2-3 carrots, large, finely shredded

Method

Preheat oven to 350°F. Grease and flour a 9" x 13" baking pan.

Mix first three ingredients together and beat for approximately two minutes. Blend the dry Ingredients (the flour, baking powder, allspice and salt) well and add to the egg mixture. Add the pineapple and carrots and stir by hand to incorporate it all.

Pour the mixture into the pan and bake for 40-45 minutes or until a toothpick inserted in center comes out clean. Let cool thoroughly before icing. Use your favorite icing but add a little mint extract.

Molten Chocolate Lava Cake Recipe

Ingredients

6 tablespoons margarine

3 squares bittersweet chocolate, cut into pieces

1/2 cup sugar

6 tablespoons all-purpose flour

Pinch salt

2 eggs

2 egg yolks

1/4 teaspoon vanilla

Icing sugar, optional

Method

Line the bottoms of 4 ramekins or small custard cups with a circle of waxed paper. Grease the ramekins and set them aside.

In a medium microwavable bowl, microwave butter (or margarine) and chocolate on Hi power about 45 seconds or until chocolate is melted; stir until smooth. Whisk in sugar, flour and salt until blended. Beat in eggs, egg yolks and vanilla. Spoon even amounts into the prepared ramekins.

Cover and refrigerate 1 hour or until ready to bake (up to 24 hours).

When ready to bake, preheat oven to 450°F.

Bake for 13-15 minutes or until the edges are firm, but the centers are still slightly soft. (Do not over bake) Let cool on wire racks for 5 minutes.

To serve, carefully run a sharp knife around the cake edges. Unmold onto serving plates and remove the waxed paper.

Butter Tart Recipe

Ingredients

1 cup raisins

1/2 cup butter, or margarine

1 cup brown sugar

1 cup corn syrup

1/2 teaspoon salt

1 teaspoon vanilla

2 eggs, lightly beaten

18 tart shells, unbaked, homemade or frozen

Method

Preheat oven to 450°F.

In heavy saucepan, combine the raisins, butter, sugar, syrup and salt. Heat on a warm stove at low heat until butter is melted and the mixture is warm. Remove from heat and add vanilla and eggs. Spoon the filling into the tart shells.

Bake for 10 minutes. Reduce heat to 350°F and bake for 5 minutes or longer until pastry is golden. Do not let the pastry filling bubble. Let butter tarts cool completely before removing from the tart tin.

German Chocolate Cake Recipe

Ingredients

4 ounces baking chocolate, sweet German

1/2 cup water

2 cups sugar

1 cup butter, softened

4 eggs, large

2 1/4 cups all-purpose flour, or 2 1/2 cups cake flour

1 teaspoon baking soda

1 teaspoon salt

1 teaspoon vanilla

1 cup buttermilk

Frosting:

1 cup sugar

1/2 cup butter

1 cup evaporated milk

1 teaspoon vanilla

3 egg yolks

1 1/3 cups flaked coconut

1 cup pecans, chopped

Method

Heat oven to 350ºF.

Grease the bottom and sides of 3 round pans that are either 8" or 9" round by 1 1/2" deep. Line the bottoms of the pans with waxed paper or cooking parchment paper.

Heat the chocolate and water in a 1 quart saucepan over low heat, stirring until the chocolate is melted.

Beat the sugar and margarine in a medium bowl with an electric mixer on high speed until light and fluffy. Beat in the eggs, one at a time. Beat in the chocolate and vanilla on low speed. Add the remaining ingredients. Beat on low speed just until blended.

Pour into two baking pans. Bake 8 inch rounds 35-40 minutes or 9 inch rounds 30-35 minutes, or until a toothpick inserted in the center comes out clean.

Cool for 10 minutes then remove from pans to a wire rack. Remove the paper and cool completely.

To Make the Frosting:

Mix the sugar, margarine, milk, vanilla and egg yolks in a 2 quart saucepan. Cook over medium heat for 12 minutes, stirring occasionally, until thick. Stir in the coconut and pecans. Cool for 30 minutes, beating occasionally, until the mixture is spreadable.

Fill the layers and frost the top of the cake with the frosting, leaving the sides of the cake unfrosted.

Dark Fruit Cake

Ingredients

2 cups Sultana raisins

2 cups seedless raisins

1 1/2 cups currants

1 1/2 cups candied cherries, halved

1 1/2 cups mixed candied fruit

1 1/2 cups chopped dates

1 1/2 cups pecans, halves

1 cup apples, finely chopped pared and cored

2 3/4 cups all-purpose flour

1 teaspoon baking powder

1 1/2 teaspoons cinnamon

1 1/2 teaspoons ginger

1 1/2 teaspoons mace

1 teaspoon ground cloves

1/2 teaspoon salt

1 cup butter

1 cup brown sugar, firmly packed

6 eggs

1/4 cup light molasses

2 squares, 2 ounces unsweetened chocolate, melted

Method

Line a 9" or 10" tube pan with two thicknesses of buttered brown paper.

Combine the fruits, nuts and fresh apple in a large bowl. Dredge the fruit with 1/4 cup of the flour.

Measure 2 1/2 cups flour (without sifting) onto a square of waxed paper. Add baking powder, spices and salt. Stir well to blend.

Cream together butter and brown sugar until light and fluffy. Add eggs one at a time, beating well after each addition. Beat in molasses and melted chocolate.

Add blended dry ingredients to creamed mixture, combining well. Stir in fruit and nut mixture until well mixed.

Spread batter evenly in prepared pan.

Preheat oven to 275°F.

Bake for about 2 1/2 hours, or until a cake tester inserted in the center comes out clean. Let the cake cool completely in the pan on a wire rack. Remove cake from the pan, peel off paper and wrap in foil. Store in an airtight container or in refrigerator for several weeks.

To Glaze and Decorate Cake - Combine 1 cup sugar, 1/2 cup water and 1/3 cup light corn syrup in a sauce pan. Stir over low heat until sugar is dissolved, then boil to firm ball stage (242°F on a candy thermometer).

Brush hot glaze over cooled cake. Decorate the top with candied cherries and nuts and brush cake again with hot glaze. Let dry thoroughly before wrapping and storing.

Graham Cracker Crust Recipe

Ingredients

1 1/2 cups graham crackers, regular or cinnamon, finely crushed

1/3 cup butter, or margarine, melted

3 tablespoons sugar

Method

Heat the oven to 350°F.

Mix the crumbs, margarine and sugar. Press the mixture firmly against the bottom and side of a pie plate, 9" x 1 1/4". Bake for 10 minutes or until light brown.

Cool before filling the pie shell.

Apple Pie Recipe

Ingredients

1 double pie crust recipe, you will find 2 recipes here

5 to 6 cups apples, peeled and thinly sliced

1/2 to 3/4 cup sugar, to your taste and depends on the sweetness of the apples

3 tablespoons flour

1 to 1 1/2 teaspoons cinnamon

1 dash salt

2 tablespoons butter, cold

Method

Preheat the oven to 425ºF.

Lay 1/2 the pastry, rolled out to about 1/8" thickness, in the bottom of the pie pan and press it in gently to lay flat in the pan. Leave the excess crust hanging over the edges for now.

Place peeled, sliced apples in a bowl. Mix together the sugar, flour, salt and cinnamon. Pour over sliced apples and mix. Fill the pie pan with the apples and pat down with a spoon. Dot the filling with pieces of butter.

Moisten the lip of the pie pan with water. Place the top layer of rolled out crust over the filling, making sure crust reaches outer edges of the pie pan all around. Seal the edge and flute all around (see notes below for how to flute a pie edge).

Take a fork and prick the pie top in several places to create vents for steam to escape. Bake for 50 minutes, until pastry is golden and the filling is bubbling through the vents.

Let cool a bit before cutting to allow the filling to settle.

Soft Chocolate Chip Cookie Recipe with Blueberries

Ingredients

1/4 cup butter, cubed, plus extra for greasing

3/4 cup all-purpose flour

1 1/2 teaspoon baking powder

1 teaspoon ground cinnamon

1/3 cup brown sugar

1/2 cup milk

1/2 cup blueberries, fresh

1/4 cup white chocolate chips

Method

Preheat the oven to 375°F.

Lightly grease a large baking sheet.

Sift the flour, baking powder, and cinnamon into a bowl. Rub in the butter or margarine, using your fingertips, until the mixture resembles rough bread crumbs, then stir in the sugar.

Stir in the milk, blueberries, and chocolate chips until just combined (the dough will be quite sticky}. Spoon 8 mounds, spaced well apart, onto the baking sheet and bake for 20 minutes at 375°F, or until golden and springy to the touch.

Cool on a wire rack for a few minutes before serving.

Chocolate Coconut Bar Cookie

Ingredients

1/2 cup butter

1 1/2 cups graham cracker crumbs

14 ounces sweetened condensed milk, 1 can

6 ounce semi-sweet chocolate chips

1 1/3 cups flaked coconut

1 cup chopped nuts

Method

Preheat oven to 350°F.

Melt butter in a 9"x13" baking pan. Sprinkle crumbs over butter. Pour sweetened condensed milk evenly over crumbs. Sprinkle chocolate chips. Coconut and nuts evenly over the top. Press down lightly.

Bake for 25 to 30 minutes until lightly browned. When cold, cut into bars.

No Bake Cookies with Chocolate Coating

Ingredients

2 cups sugar

1/3 cup cocoa

1/2 cup butter

1/2 cup milk

1/2 cup peanut butter

1 teaspoon vanilla

3 cups rolled oats, quick-cooking

Method

Combine sugar, cocoa, butter and milk in saucepan. Bring to a boil. Boil 1 minute. Remove from heat and stir in the peanut butter until melted, then add vanilla and oats.

Drop by spoonful onto waxed paper and allow to harden.

Lemon Tarts

Ingredients

2 cups flour

1/2 teaspoon salt

2/3 cup shortening

5-6 tablespoons cold water

1/2 cup butter, or margarine

1 cup sugar

1 tablespoon cornstarch

3 eggs, beaten

1/2 cup lemon juice

Method

Preheat oven to 400°F.

For the shells, combine the flour and salt. Cut in the shortening with a pastry blender until the mixture resembles coarse meal. Sprinkle cold water evenly over the surface.

Stir with a fork until all the dry ingredients are moistened. Shape the dough into a ball and chill.

When chilled, roll the dough to 1/8 inch thickness on a lightly floured surface. Cut into 3 1/4 inch rounds. Fit each pastry round into 3 inch tart pans. Prick with a fork.

Bake in a preheated oven for 10-12 minutes. Let cool.

Place the butter in the top of a double boiler. Bring the water in the double boiler to a boil. Reduce the heat to low, and cook until the butter melts. Combine the sugar and cornstarch, stirring well. Add to the butter and stir until smooth. Stir in the eggs and cook for 5 minutes, stirring constantly.

Add the lemon juice. Cook 3-4 minutes longer or until the mixture thickens, stirring constantly. Cool. Spoon a rounded tablespoon of lemon filling into each cooled tart shell.